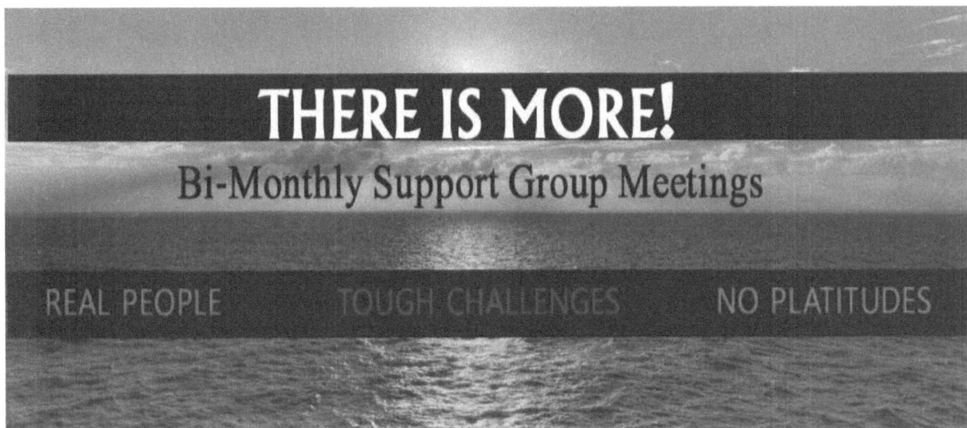

ThereIsMoreMeeting.Com

A support Group that reaches to the
Body, Mind and Soul

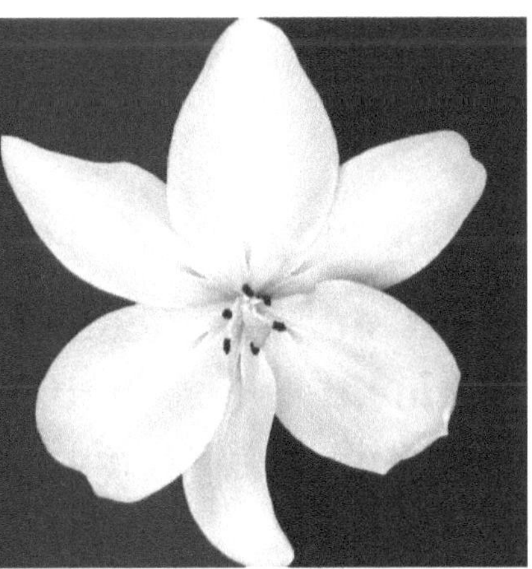

Tom's Nuero Notes

A collection of blogs Tom Schuck.

Not intended as medical advice, but as anecdotal and situational understanding from personal experience and observing and listening to others.

Contents

First Day, Now What?

Before I begin Anything else, I have three core thoughts that I want you to keep in mind from here on.

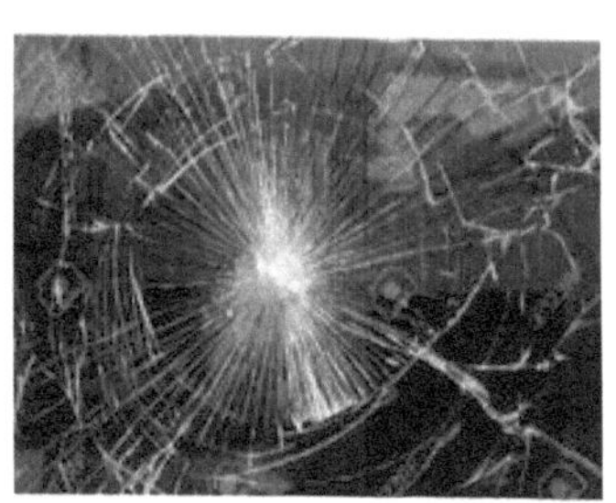

You are NOT ALONE.

THIS is going to be a journey.

You are not alone, there are countless families, individuals, young children, middle age workers, and elderly post-retirees who are stepping off on the journey this very day, or are much farther down the road than you will want to imagine right now.

THIS is going to be a journey.

This is the beginning of your journey, not the ending of it. Strokes and Brain injuries are very, very dangerous, and neither your doctor, nor your medical care team will want to speculate on hope during the first few days.

But I deal in hope. I have heard countless stories of survivors, and I am one of them.

There is More, a whole "new" you to be uncovered

Like Dr. Steven Strange who thought he lost everything when he lost his ability to be a brilliant neurosurgeon, he found his new meaning in as a Marvel Superhero

Be ready to accept that which was the "old you" and that which is the "new you"

You could come out of this completely unscathed. Many do. Many others discover that there will be changes: Abilities and activities that they can no longer do, will be replaced by new passions, new activities, based on new abilities.

For some, this interruption of your life, will end up being no more than a "stay in the hospital" and you will go home with little to no residuals, but for many others it will mark the 1st day of who you will be, and all that you WILL do, what every survivor calls "the OLD me and the NEW me".

<u>Your Support Team</u>

From Day 1, Your Support Team will Consist of 3 Elements, which we will explore in detail in this book:

- Your First team member in your recovery process is knowledge. What happened to you, what will happen to you.

- After you leave hospital care you will want to know where and who you will turn to for medical treatment and advice

- Last, but certainly not least in importance, will be finding local and on-line support groups, discussing your experiences with others who have been on the survivor's journey for months or years.

Why are these so important?

If you are still in the hospital, or in full time physical therapy, there will come time,

      much sooner than you or your family feel is appropriate

         that you will be released back home to finish your recovery.

When this happens, you will feel UNPREPARED and INSUFFICIENTLY INFORMED to navigate "what I am supposed to do next?"

I also need to state unapologetically, that I am not a trained medical professional. I am a survivor, and a leader of two support groups. I am also a very good listener. I also spend hours reading and 'listening' to stories of survivors on Facebook websites. I am also, whenever I can be, an advocate for survivors.

All the evidence that I have is 100% anecdotal. This means that it comes from real people, current people, talking about how they feel in support groups and online groups. I wish that the medical profession would utilize more anecdotal evidence in their treatment and understanding of the survivor.

Your Physicians and Specialists were there to protect your life and return you back to a state of physical stasis. They were not, and are not there to advise you on how to be a person again. After all, a brain injury or stroke is one of the, if not, the MOST, life shattering injuries that can happen to a person.

So, let's look at what happens next!

<u>Knowledge</u>

Modern neurologists do not often use the work stroke or brain injury in a hospital clinical setting. Most often the immediate diagnosis is "CVA" for "Cerebral Vascular Accident" or "Blood Vessel Accident in the area of the brain".

Medical society divides this into several types. For ease of understanding, I have simplified the chart to the following.

- ABI: Acquired Brain Injury.
  - ABI:STROKE – due to poor health
  - ABI:BIRTH – Birth defect issues
  - ABI:ABI – caused by heart attack, medical procedure, etc.

  - TBI: Traumatic Brain Injury
    - TBI: Force Impact
    - TBI: Dissected Artery – Whiplash, over twisting of vertebral artery

  - Hemorrhagic bleeding

Although stroke is prevalent in those with high risk heart disease, my anecdotal experience is that most patients are admitted due to some form of TBI, of which VAD or Vertebral Arterial Dissection (especially among young people 15-35) is growing at an alarming rate.

March 23, 2018 <u>admin</u> <u>Stroke</u>, <u>stroke support</u>, <u>TBI</u> Comments Off

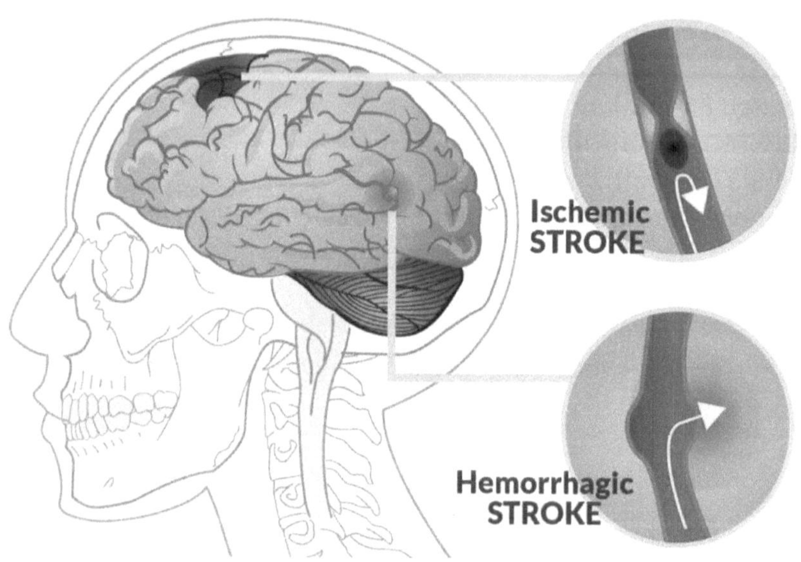

Stroke.Org and several other major medical organizations have developed the symptom recognition tool called FAST. But recently, a new general symptom for recognizing that a stroke is imminent has been added.
First, what is Fast?

Well Now, it seems that the T is Fast should be replaced to stand for the TONGUE.

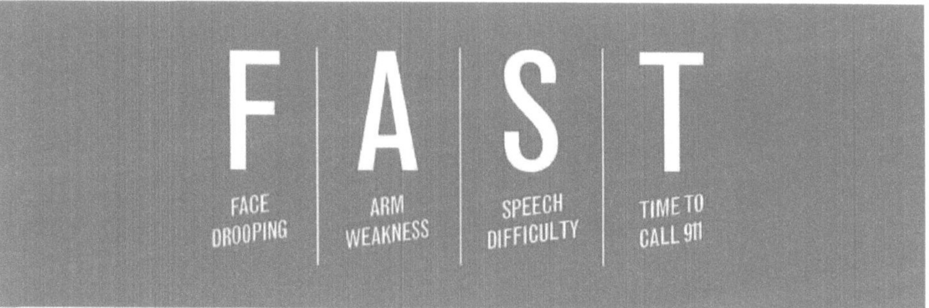

For example, If you, or a suspected person, falls for no good reason, or excuses it as a "new shoe" or "bum knee" ask them to humor you and stick out their tongue. If the tongue is crooked to one side rather than straight, THIS MAY INDICATE A STROKE.

Another example. If you or a suspected person is complaining of numbness on one side of their body, you may also want to apply the tongue check, or the entire fast routine.

F A S T E R

Is Face vDropping	Can they raise both <u>arms</u> and be level	Can they SMILE	Tongue is crooked to one side	Get them to the ER now
	Ask them complex questions that they should know?	Speach Difficulty		

So I have developed the FastER code.

F: Is their Face drooping on one side?

A: can stand for either "Arms", can they evenly raise both arms. "A" also stands for "Ask". Ask the person a moderately difficult question that they should know the answer to.

S: Can stand for either "Smile". is one side of the smile drooped? Or "S" can stand for "speech difficulty", are they mumbling or not making sense?

T: Now stands for Tongue. Stick it out. Is it crooked or straight?

ER: I added this to stand for: get the person to the ER. You have an emergency on your hands.

Calling all VADers

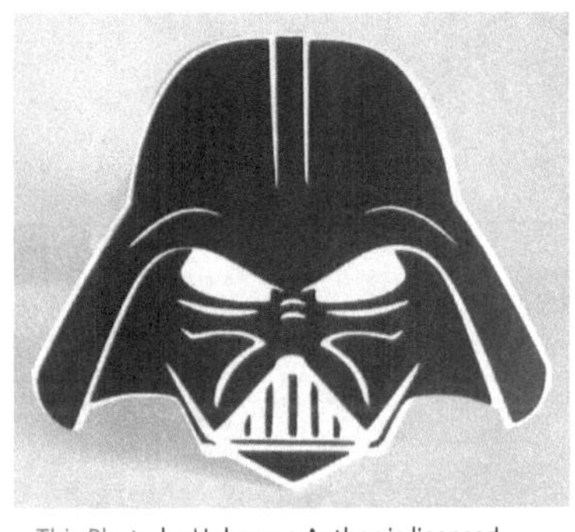

No, **not Darth Vader**, but LVADers and RVADers. This is an growing epidemic of "stroke" among young people, striking teenagers and 40 year old fit and trim individuals alike. One Facebook group, _Vertebral Arterial Support Group_ has 2,200 members and is growing at the rate of nearly 30 per month. Another group, _Wallenburg or Lateral Medullary Syndrome Group_, which covers one of the more painful, lasting effects of VAD currently has just over 350 members.

So what is VAD? VAD stands for Vertebral Arterial Dissection. Which means, "leading into the brain and brainstem, an Artery (not a Vein), has been (On the inside wall of the arterial) split open". This causes an "occlusion", BAD thing, a stoppage of flow to the brain.

Mechanically, what happens is that the VAD occurs as an injury (TBI, Traumatic brain injury), often without the person knowing it. A sudden twisting of the neck, and the inner lining of the artery tears away forming a pocket, behind which blood will seep through and clot.

Vertebral Artery Dissection With development of Cerebral Infarct

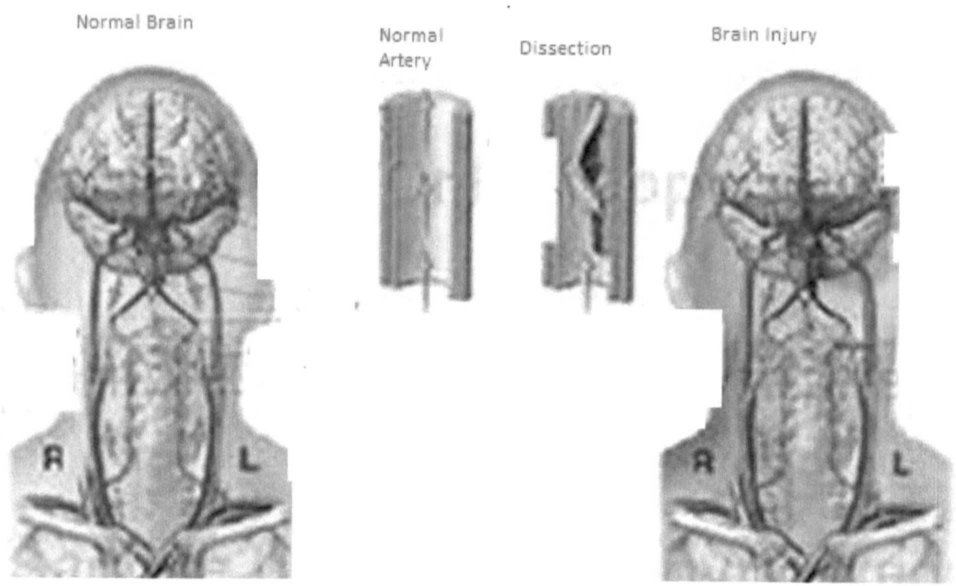

Sometimes attributed to side impact crashes, whiplash, Neck Adjustment, Dancing and floor sports where the technique of "spotting" is used. (Spotting in dance is when the dance partner or athlete maintains their head facing one direction, then turns their body as far as possible without moving their head, and finally rapidly whips their head back to original position). Officially on medical charts, my LVAD (Left Arterial Vertebral Dissection) cause was listed as "Ballroom Dancing".

The first symptom that an individual often reports is serious migraine-type headaches for weeks or months, even though the individual is not prone to headaches.

The second symptom, which can occur weeks or months afterwards, is that the torn lining gives way in the artery and a rush of lining debris, clotted blood and blood rush into the medulla and brain. This is felt as a shock of dizziness and uneasiness.

In a fraction of a second, the individual is suffering a complete stroke, the final symptom of the VAD.

For me, I was ballroom dancing when the stroke occurred. I have no idea what I was doing when the original injury occurred. The good part was that my headaches finally ended. But my long journey from victim to encouraging survivor was just beginning. Typical of strokes was the loss of walking, speech, eye coordination, balance. Atypical was the amount of awareness and cognitive abilities I maintained. I was rattled, but not confused. I lost the mental ability to add two numbers together, but not to understand the significance of numbers on a spreadsheet.

I was also surprised how quickly I progressed, but for VADers, this is also not unusual. With good physical therapy, I was walking with a cane, communicating clearly, and even able to drive within 35 days.

All of these are normal progressions for the VADers. Later, unfortunately, I was in the 40% that does not recover fully. After 1 and ½ years, a series of setbacks and minor strokes reversed many of my advances, removing my ability to drive or work, and put me permanently walking with a cane.

I

Some survivors of a Vertebral Arterial Dissection may go on to live life with some degree of Lateral Medullary Syndrome.

Also called "Wallenbergs Syndrome" this syndrome is not limited to survivors of brain injury alone, but for the purpose of this booklet, that is the only area being discussed.

Signs and symptoms

- This syndrome is characterized by
- Sensory deficits that affect the trunk and extremities contralaterally.
    - If your injury was on the left side of your brain, your right side will have sensory deficits.
    - Conversely you can tell which side of the brain was affected by noticing which side of your body (from your shoulders down) has sensory deficits.
- Deficits include lack of feeling HOT, COLD, PINCH from a needle, PIN or nail.
- General Lower body temperature
- Lower Strength and coordination
- Loss of 'tickle effect'

- One oddity is the deficit generally shifts sides at your neck and affects various spots all over your face and head, favoring the opposite side of your body deficits.
- Balance and difficulty walking, wide gait, fear of steps, over-leaning to one side or the other.
    - Many of these are vestibular, Nystagmus (eye-shaking), eyes not teaming, or pupils dilated at different sizes.

- o Other balance issues are a combination of vestibular and damage to the balance center of the brain.
- Nucleus ambiguus - (which affects vagus nerve and glossopharyngeal nerve) - dysphagia, hoarseness, absent gag reflex
  - o Difficulty Swallowing
- Maintaining full intellectual skills, but having severe difficult expressing intellect through speech. Often out performs at writing, but can be very insecure in speaking.

- Constant 24/7 pain, mostly through affected side. Although nerves have become insensitive to most external stimuli (handling a hot cup, feeling a cut or impalement), the nerves appear to be in a constant and painful misfire of their own.

- Mood swings and emotional outburst (crying, anger) due to damage to the amygdala)

According to Wikipedia, lateral medullary syndrome is the most common form of posterior ischemic stroke syndrome. They estimated around 600,000 new cases of this syndrome in the United States alone

Medical Staff

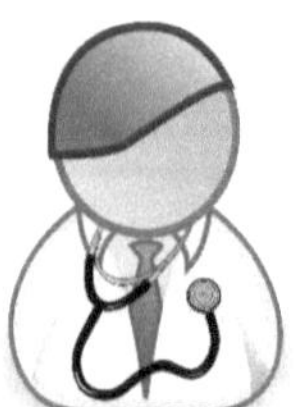

✓ Treats: All your medical needs.
✓ Likely to defer Neurological treatment to your Neurologist
✓ See: 1 to 4 visits per year
✓ Prescribes

Primary Care Physician

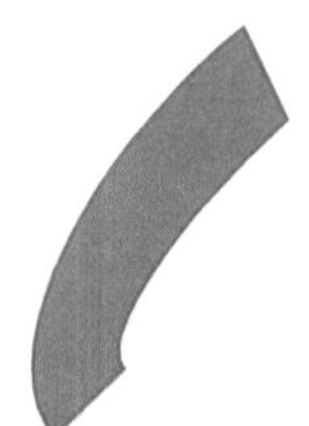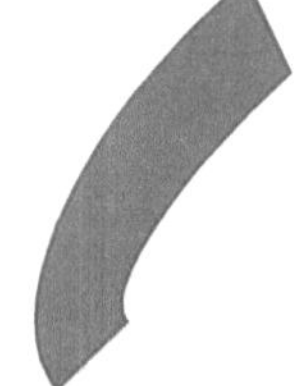

✓ Treats: Monitors stability 1-3 years
✓ See: 3 to 4 visits first 1-2 years.
✓ See: 1 to 2 visits thereafter
✓ Prescribes

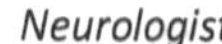

Neurologist

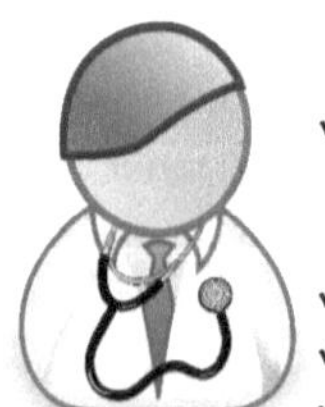

✓ Treats: brain, vascular health. "coach for the brain". Most include PT
✓ See: 3 to 4 visits per year
✓ Prescribes
✓ When not available, may be replaced by Neurophyscologist.

Neurophysiatrist

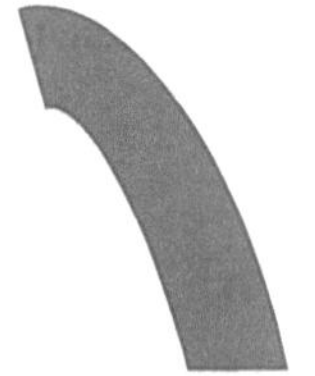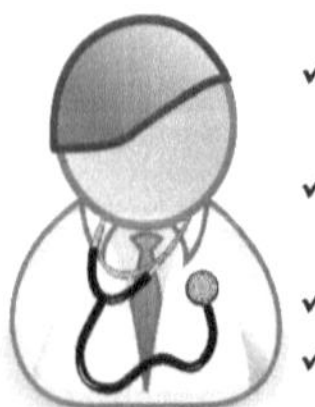

Role of your Primary Care Doctor.

Your current PMP doctor is still your primary warehouse of your complete medical history. Even though he probably will not actively engage in testing your recovery process or post brain injury/stroke skills. Making sure that every other Doctor, Physical Therapist or testing lab sends a copy of their activity and report to your PMP is vital to make sure that your doctor knows how to distinguish between a symptom of your brain injury and any other symptoms of medical need in your body.

Role of your Neurologist.

Immediately following your return to home, your neurologist will probably want to see you at the 3, 6, 9 and 12 month mark. Maybe less , if you are progressing. Following that, your visits will decline to twice a year, then once a year.

Your Appointment.

- ✓ It's best to bring another person with you into the room to listen to the neurologist, and **take notes**. Your neurologist may say many things that you may want to look up later, some that may even unnerve you at first. Having another, somewhat impartial set of ears will be of great benefit to you.

What should you tell your neurologist?

- ✓ ALL your medications, prescribed and over the counter vitamins.
- ✓ All your symptoms, including hiccups, increased nightmares, difficulty swallowing, pain, vision problems, Everything. Don't leave out any details. BE YOUR OWN ADVOCATE!!!

What will your neurologist do?

- ✓ Prescribe medications based on how you emphasize your symptoms.
- ✓ Perform basic neurological function tests, such as following a pencil with your eyes, touching your nose with your fingers, standing still with eyes closed, and the like.

<u>Role of your Neurophysiatrist.</u>

And Neuro-Psychologist,

Soon after your relationship with your neurologist starts to extend to semi-annual or annually, you will probably want to add someone to oversee detailed items and the "physical re-training" of your brain. That is precisely the role of the Neurophysiatrist, and Neuro-psychologist.

 The Neurophysiatrist acts like a "coach for your brain". Generally these doctors spend much more time with their patients and take time to answer questions and describe answers in clear understandable detail. They also can refer to visual, speech, balance, and all sorts of other physical trainers that may even work from their own office, or nearby. The Neurophysiatrist often specializes in quality of life.

<u>Your Appointment.</u>

- ✓ It's best to bring another person into the room to help you remember what you want to say, and **<u>take notes</u>**. Your Neurophysiatrist may give you information that you will want to look up later. Having another, somewhat impartial set of ears will be of great benefit to you.

<u>What should you tell your neurophysiatrist?</u>

- ✓ ALL your medications, prescribed and over the counter vitamins.
- ✓ All your symptoms, including hiccups, increased nightmares, difficulty swallowing, pain, vision problems, Everything. Don't leave out any details
- ✓ Discuss with your Neurophysiatrist those symptoms that are impacting your quality of life, as your doctor will be most interested in solving quality of life issues.

<u>What will your Neurophysiatrist do?</u>

- ✓ Prescribe medications based on how you emphasize your symptoms.
- ✓ Ask you about your quality of life, and offer recommendations on improving.
- ✓ Recommend physical therapy for muscle or vestibular issues.
- ✓ Perform basic neurological function tests, such as following a pencil with your eyes, touching your nose with your fingers, standing still with eyes closed, and the like.

Support Groups

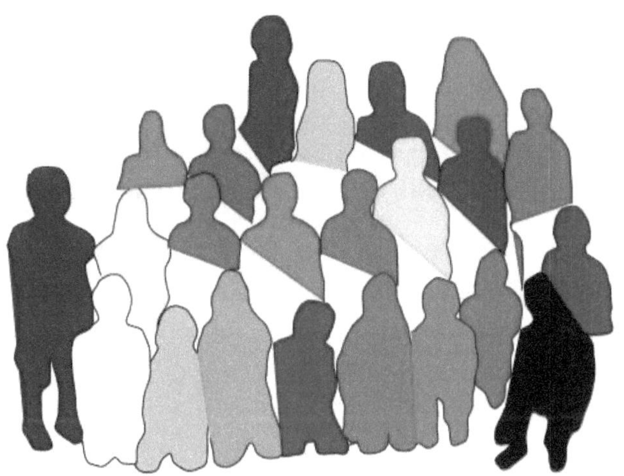

You will likely have a difficult time navigating your new life without a support group. First of all, you are on, or just beginning a journey. Each step of the journey will become heavier and heavier without having someone understand you without patronizing you or telling you to get it, or offering you one of many insulting clichés.

In a support group, no one is going to ridicule you for any symptom that you have. Believe me, I have seen and heard it all, and in our support groups, all symptoms are "normal".

Drooler, Mumbler, The One who Forgets every other word, The one who is forgetful after 20 seconds. It's all normal.

The person with no physical external markings, but marked with pain, dizziness and confusion inside, and hates to be told "You look good". It's all normal

I am currently facilitating two support groups in north central Connecticut, in Bloomfield and Manchester. Although I bring along a weekly small group curriculum every meeting, it is seldom used, as more often the attendees will come with subjects that are important, relevant and needs to be talked through now.

And, wonderfully, the whole group responds with ideas, counter ideas and lots of great discussion. When each session is done, everyone has learned, grown and written down something useful for themselves.

Support groups are NOT limited to just the "in-person". There on many on Facebook.

ThereIsMoreMeeting, Young Stroke Survivors, Second Chance Stroke Survivors and Brain Injury Awareness are 4 excellent groups to consider on Facebook.

If you are in Hartford CT on the 2nd or 4th Fridays, check out: ThereIsMoreMeeting.Com

<u>**Brain Injury Alliance of America**</u>

https://www.biausa.org/

Brain Injury Alliance of America is the political / legal awareness group and information awareness center. Most individuals interact through individual chapters. There are generally 1 or more chapters in most states.

Alaska:	https://alaskabraininjury.net/
Arizona	https://www.biaaz.org/
California	http://www.biacal.org/
Connecticut	http://www.biact.org/
Florida	https://www.biaf.org/
Illinois	https://www.biail.com/
Indiana	https://biaindiana.org/
Iowa:	https://biaia.org/
Massachusettes	http://www.biama.org/
New Jersey	https://bianj.org/
New York	https://bianys.org/
Texas	http://www.texasbia.org/
Washington	https://www.biawa.org/
Wyoming	http://www.wybia.org/

Facebook Support Groups

This is NOT a complete list of all support groups specific to stroke, brain injury, or specific symptoms.

ThereISMoreMeeting" – General, All brain Injury. Only 24 Members. Facebook group is an introduction to the group's website. Several publications available. *"Thereismoremeeting.com"*

Young Stroke Survivors – Very Active stroke and brain injury group. Active and meaningful postings. 7700 + members

Second Change Stroke Survivors – Active Stroke and Brain injury group. Active and meaningful postings. 2600+ members

TBI Survivors and Caregivers support group. Active Brain injury group. Active and meaningful postings 12000+ members

Vertebral Artery Dissection Support – Specific to those who had the Vertebral Arterial Dissection TBI/Stroke. 2400+ Members

wallenberg's syndrome or lateral medullary syndrome – Group Specific - 415+ members

How can Others help?

It is nothing like when your body gets tired, it is more like suddenly hitting a physical / emotional / psychological _**wall**_ all at once. You will need to rest, and rest now. Although survivors are not excluded from activities, they often find themselves having to curtail the time or energy expended at an activity.

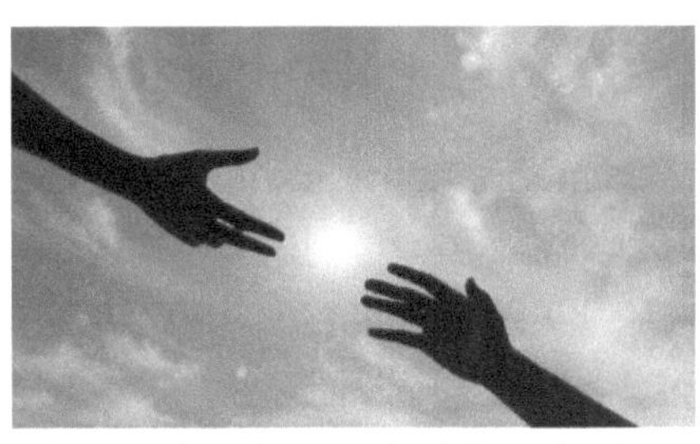

Good news. There are identifiable situations that you can avoid that may overstimulate your brain.

1. Reduce bright lights. If bright light is exhausting to your recovering brain, you may have already discovered this by your desire for dark room and darker sun glasses. Here are some additional ways you can adapt your environment:
   a. Instead of bright artificial lighting, you can try filtered sun-light through a window with blinds or drapes
   b. Wear sunglasses indoors and out. Don't worry about looking too cool.
   c. Reduce the brightness of your computer, laptop or tablet screen.
2. Remove yourself from noisy conversations. If you find that being in the presence of hearing multiple conversations taking place at one time in near proximity overtaxes your brain:
   a. Always bring along ear plugs
   b. Sit in the corner of a room, restaurant or meeting hall, so that you are not surrounded by sound sources.
   c. Offer alternatives to overcrowded venues: If you find that being in large crowded situations overtaxes your brain you can offer your suggestions for less crowded venues whenever plans are being made.

Be Your Own Advocate

In so many situations, you will have to be your own advocate. The first job of being your own advocate is to hopefully pass off that job to someone else that you can trust.

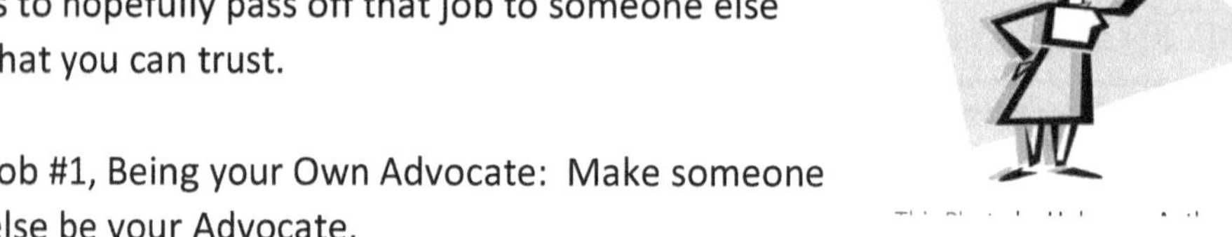

Job #1, Being your Own Advocate: Make someone else be your Advocate.

There may need to be an honest sit down discussion with your family, spouse, loved-one, partner, special person that makes them aware of certain elements of your recovery. You may work out some key phrases like:

1. My brain gets tired quickly, I cannot stay out as long as we used to. If we go out, and I do WANT to go with you, we just might have to leave early.
2. If I come up to you while we are at an event or outing, and I say "I need to go now", please understand that I am trying to avoid being noticed, but please, as quickly as possible wrap up what you are doing, and get me home.
3. I may say, I am going to sit in the car, or something like that. This means that you don't have to follow me, just know that I am taking time to rest. If people ask where I am, just brush it off, please.

Extra Notes for the Journey

(Not all notes will apply to your personal journey. See
TherelsMoreMeeting.Com for new notes being added frequently)

"It's Not Character, its Chemical"

Too many survivors receive damage to their amygdala and other critical emotion control and hormone emitting centers of the brain. When these areas of the brain are damaged you will find that your "character" is changing in ways that is abnormal for you. You may become weepy, sullen, depressed, or filled with rage. You may be filled with fear that your family is now Enemy #1 in your life. You may be convinced that your spouse is out to harm you.

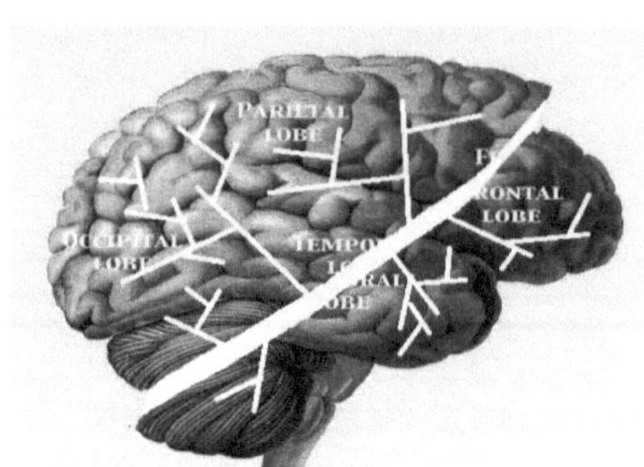

All of these derive from areas of the brain that have been damaged and are not emitting, or emitting to much of the proper hormonal substances that are necessary to equalize our temperament and reactions.

Don't fear the Psychologist, or Neurologist, who steps in and starts prescribing "psych" drugs to take the place of those that your brain cannot emit.

Just because you are taking these "Pysch" drugs DOES NOT MEAN that you have a mental illness, or are in any way mentally ill because of your brain injury or stroke. It simply means that you require a little therapy to overcome any losses that your body is NOT PRODUCING.

I am on the very gentle, dual purpose pain and pysch medication, Cymbalta. I will be taking these for the foreseeable future. Whenever I miss a dosage, I start to view my loving wife of 35+ years as the wicked witch of the east. When I am level of the medication, my mind, actions and marriage are normal, with all the normal stuff that couples face.

<u>Why didn't they tell me?</u>

- Your brain is going to get tired. , don't be ashamed of the need of the desire for frequent daytime catnaps.
- Don't be ashamed or stop your social life, BUT DO explain your limitations. To your Date or spouse, explain, "I love to go out for the evening, but my brain tires easily and I may need to leave early", or "Can we sit in the corner away from the noise?".
- You may have spent a good part of your life supporting others, caring for others, leading others. Those people had to accept your gift of care and support. It is your turn now to accept help from others. Let others feel good for being able to help you.
- Violent day-long hiccups are the norm for many survivors, as well as a little choking on food, spitting up, and difficulty swallowing. This is due to the deadening of vital nerve responses around the esophagus.
- It is not abnormal for some of your friends to have a problem coping with your changes. Their inability to cope is not a reflection on your relationship, it is merely how they are wired to handle trauma in their lives, which is not very good. Many friends will disappear because you cannot offer the level of entertainment and friendship that they always knew.
- The more highly specialized your physician, the more likely he/she will have what you perceive as poor bedside manners. They will seem clinical, not offering hope to you or your family, but rather making clinical observations that tend to lead your worrying mind down the darkest paths. Don't let this get to you. They are on your team.
- You need a team of care. Minimally it should consist of your PMP (Primary care physician), your Neurologist (that you eventually cut back to seeing only every 6 months to once a year), and either a Neurophysiatrist (recommended) or a Neuropsychologist.
- Your family, close friends, doctors are NOT THE ENEMY. You may often feel that they do not or cannot feel the extent of your physical pain or emotional loss, but they truly want to help.

Easter Seals: Neuro-Pysch test. Early Basis Test.

Although I had very disparaging remarks for my neuropysch exam, I would have to base the success or lack of, on the fact that the attending physician announced his unfavorable breakup with the medical company that he was testing at, before we even began.

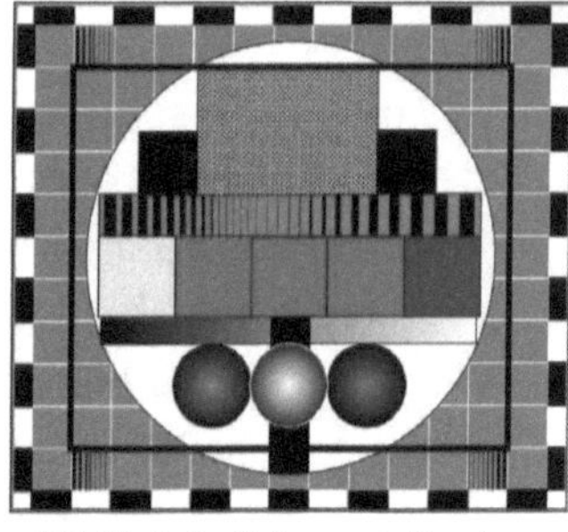

Leaving that behind, the Neuro-pysch test is your next stop, even after being pronounced well, or well-enough.

According to WebMd (https://www.webmd.com/brain/neuropsychological-test#1-2)

- If you're having trouble concentrating or making decisions, some simple tests might be helpful in figuring out what's wrong. They're called neuropsychological tests.
- Neuropsychology looks at how the health of your brain affects your thinking skills and behavior.

These tests are usually done as a combination of pencil and paper in a doctor's office, part on a computer, and part where a neuropsychologist will just ask you a series of questions that you answer orally.

What's on These Tests?

These tests help your doctors look at your attention span and how well you concentrate on things. Other areas covered by neuropsychological testing include:

- Your ability to think, understand, learn, and remember (cognition)
- <u>Memory</u>
- Motor function (walking, coordination, etc.)
- Perception (how well you take in what you see or read)
- Problem-solving and decision-making
- Verbal ability

<u>Here are some examples of the kinds of tests you might be given:</u>

- Memory test: Repeat a list of words, sentences, or numbers.
- Cognition test: Explain how two items are like. For instance, if you see a picture of a dog and a cat, you might answer that they're both animals or that they are both pets.
- Verbal communication test: Name some items as the person giving the test points at them. You might also be given a letter of the alphabet and told to list words that start with that letter.
- Motor tests: These might include tasks such as inserting pegs into a pegboard using one hand and then the other.
- You might also be given tests to see how your hearing and vision affect your thinking and memory.

When Asked "When Do I Need This Kind of Testing?

One of 4 of the primary reasons is "brain injury"

If you decide to proceed to go ahead, you should do so as early after your brain injury/stroke as possible. This is used to create a base-line, that can later with future evaluations, measure progress.

Since these tests are often given to healthy individuals, the tests are designed to be taken in 1 eight hour day.

When I took mine, fortunately my wife was there as my advocate and told them that I was incapable of sitting for eight hours.

They offered to break it down to two four-hour days. We settled for three days, three hours each. Contact your local Easter Seals for more information.

Common Symptoms that are rarely clinically documented

The Brain jolt – "Electrical lightning bolts"

A common experience of many survivors that may arise immediate or **years after** their initial event are Brain Jolts. (also sometimes called brain shivers, brain shocks, head shocks, and electrical shocks). They tend to be apparently uncaused sensations of electricity briefly passing through the brain. Some describe them as "a sudden jolt or buzz in the brain." Others report that they feel like "short bursts of white light or lightning mixed with

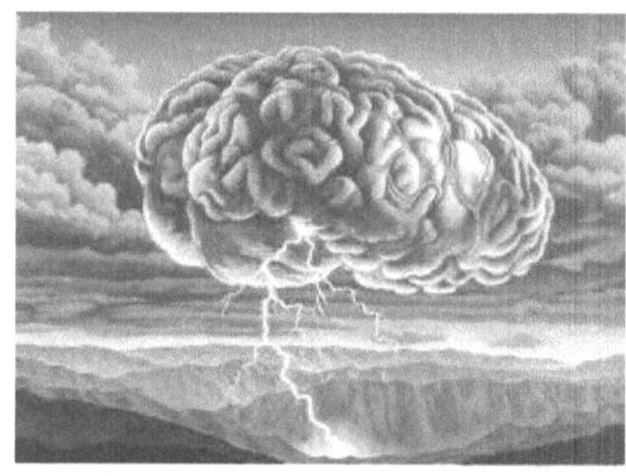

dizziness." Sometimes brain zaps are accompanied by vertigo, tinnitus, throat tension and nausea. Others will report that the attack is like a powerful discharge in the center of their brain that travels down through their body, causing the arms and legs to convulse, and the person to lose balance and possibly fall. It has been described by one observing EMT as "fully resembling a Petit Mal Seizure".

Even though you can print pages of anecdotal evidence from Facebook of people who describe these symptoms, many neurologists agree that there are too little actual clinical studies, and that the actual mechanisms are unknown. Some neurologists will suggest that you are unique, or that they never heard of such of symptom accompanying brain injury or stroke. Within the entire medical community, some won't entirely believe you, or understand your description. Others will fortunately prescribe anti-epileptic medications, which seems to reduce the quantity and violence of these events to near 0.

<u>*Sudden Super-Heated Nerve zones*</u>
Related closely to the electricity issues of Brain Jolts, this occurs when the survivor's internal control of their electrical systems have been damaged by the injury to the brain. The nervous system evidently now stores up electrical energy as heat at certain points. There have been NO anecdotal notes on this leading to any form of human combustion. Usually the patient just needs a quick temporary application of cold compress.

<u>*Knots and Bumps of Nerves bundles not found on MRI*</u>
I have two zones of these. One that is rather permanent in my center back. Sometimes, it is large and hard, other times it is soft and movable. Each time, when the lump has been at it worst, I have it x-rayed and MRI'd several times, and each time the results are negative.
It cannot be messaged out, or reduced by medications. It is a nerve bundle that Is (anecdotally) a result of brain injury.
This is a rarer symptom, I have only found a few other a few others on Facebook who identify with this symptom, and inability to cure it.

April 4, 2019 admin Stroke, stroke support, TBI Comments Off

Depression and Neurological Injuries

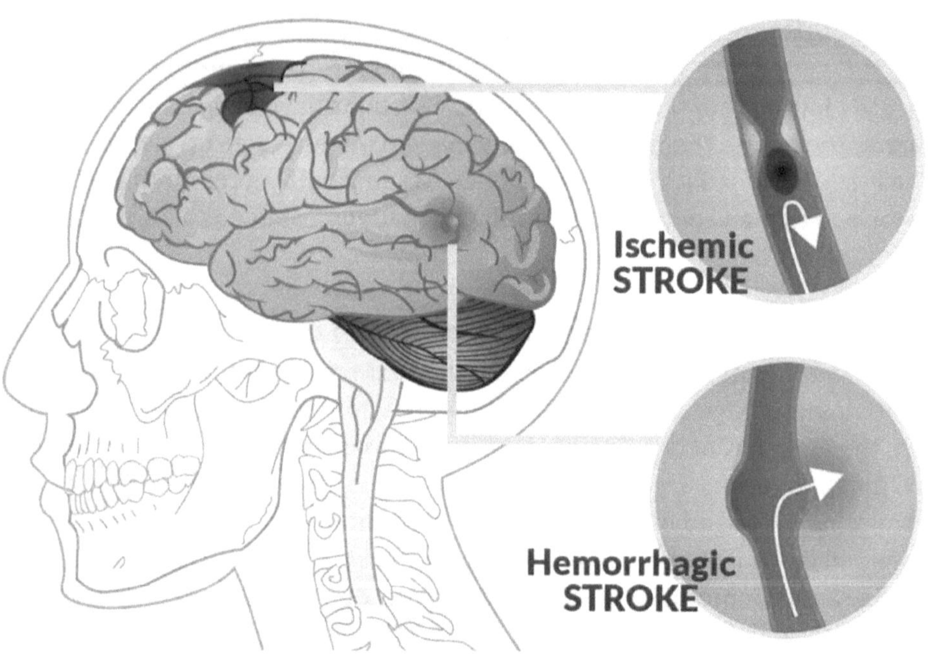

More doctors are using ketamine to treat severe depression in patients who haven't responded to other treatments.

I am not a Doctor. I am an Observer, a listener, and I share what I have gathered (without sharing confidences)

I have developed a unique view to depression, including my own depression, including that depression which leads to the handling of the artifacts of suicide, and again, including that which I 'played' with myself.

Depression, as a Neurological component IS a direct result of

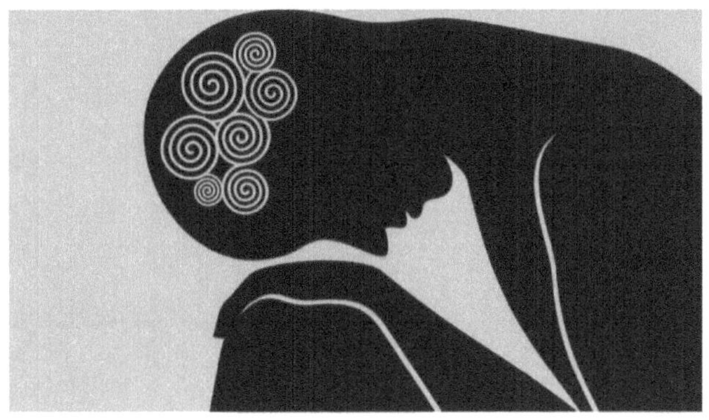

a dangerous CHEMICAL imbalance in the individual caused by partial or complete damage to those organs in the brain responsible to create and release those hormones and chemicals. They cannot be produced elsewhere in the brain or body and supplemental pharmaceuticals are required to supplement the lost activities performed by those organs.

But Depression also has an emotional aspect that I DO NOT believe that counseling alone will relieve.

This is because it is my observation that depression can be a symptom of LOSS (among other things). And the survivor of Neurological Illness and Injury has a long list of Losses to think about.

My Top 5 "Losses"

1.   Dignity - often first lost when the individual finds themselves being "cared for".

2.   Independence - often first lost by revoked or limited driving privileges, or being restricted to a wheel chair, etc.

3.   Role - Lost when the individual looses their job, or structure, especially when the survivor is forced to watch others doing the work that gave them satisfaction.

4.   Desirability - A distinct loss that occurs when the survivor is encouraged to just watch rather than engage in social activities, and becomes more evident when those who care for the survivor talk about needing a vacation from them.

5.   Memory - Memory may or may not be damaged heavily in a typical injury or illness.

<u>A Few practical solutions.</u>

1.   "Care For" must be replaced with "Cared About". I make this distinction. *Cared for* is merely the act of doing good things, checking in on the survivor, cooking, gives them their daily pills, etc. *Cares about* are the sincere actions of the heart, spending time joking, reading, talking about relevant subjects, holding hands, touching, hugging.

2.   The loss of Independence, which includes physical activities of independence, now need to be replaced with TRUST.

3.   *Roles lost* need to be replaced with *Roles given*. What can I, the survivor, be given to be responsible for?

4.   Desirability – For family members and survivors, anytime that caring and being cared for becomes a '**job**', a serious inquiry needs to made into home health care aides, or just talking about reducing tensions and expectations.

5.   Memories. Have several "old photographs" parties where the family discusses the photos and the events in each photo.

April 4, 2019 admin Stroke, stroke support, TBI Comments Off

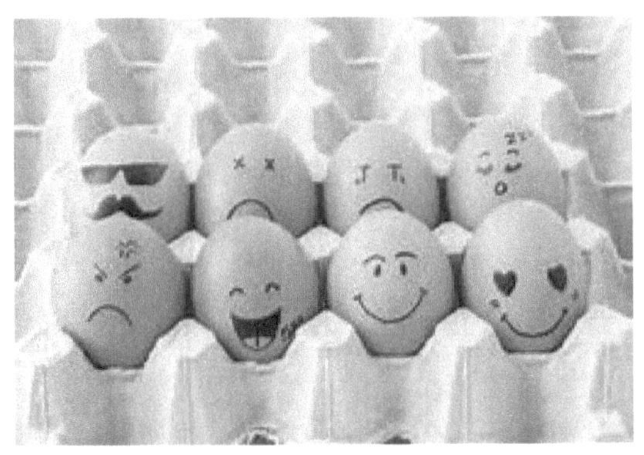

I get this question asked of me every morning, and it is perhaps the most difficult to answer, if not the most profound question of the morning. On one hand, I know that if I flippantly respond "fine", "well", then the other person expects me to act as if I feel well, when that is farthest from the truth. On the other hand, I know that NO ONE likes a complainer, and if I give too much detail, or take too much time describing how I really feel, it is the quickest way to shove people away from me.

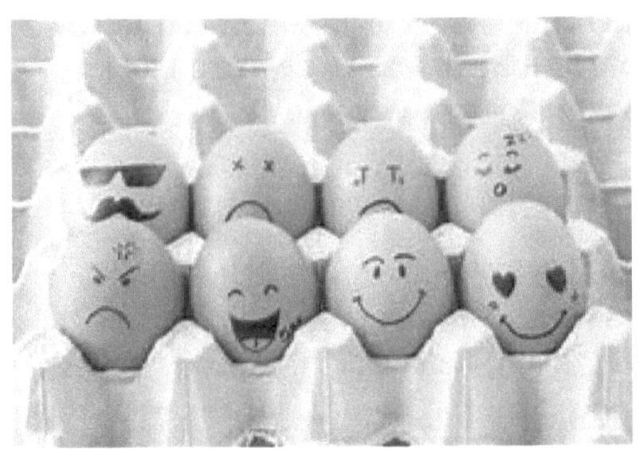

Having been a pastor and counselor before my personal brain injury, has given me a *little* insight on how to govern myself and in the process, I believe that I have stumbled on two successful ***analogies*** to answer the question **"How are you feeling today"**, honestly and accurately.

First, I have found, so far, that there are two primary types of overwhelming "Not doing well", for the brain injury and stroke survivor, they are.

1. Pain/dizziness
2. Unable to muster energy

- For Pain and dizziness, I first ask each person that will be asking me that question on a regular basis, spouse, family, close friends, doctors, etc., to recall for themselves the level of pain, dizziness, discomfort and general inability to think when they have had a 100 degree fever or more.

Then I add to that, "Now imagine yourself when you have a 102 degree fever, how would you feel; now 104 degree fever, now 106, now 108 fevers?"

After asking them to have these analogies fixed in their in head, I tell them, (This is my actual personal response) "My normal pain/dizziness NEVER drops below 102, that is what I cope with 24/7. Right now, I am about xxx degrees, I don't have a real fever, that's just how you would feel if you were me.

- **Second.** Energy Swings. It is difficult to explain the sudden "hitting the wall" effect that affects so many survivors. How one moment you feel normal and active, and suddenly, your brain shuts your entire body down. Unless you have had a near death-acceptance experience, such as near drowning or near choking or similar, I cannot come up with a similar life experience that approximates the suddenness and overwhelming shut down, sometimes accompanied by neuropathic pain.
- The fear of these episodes keeps some survivors from engaging in activities at all, rather than learning their body responses and being prepared.

Brain Injury / Stroke and the Loss of Emotions

September 8, 2018 admin Stroke, stroke support, TBI Comments Off

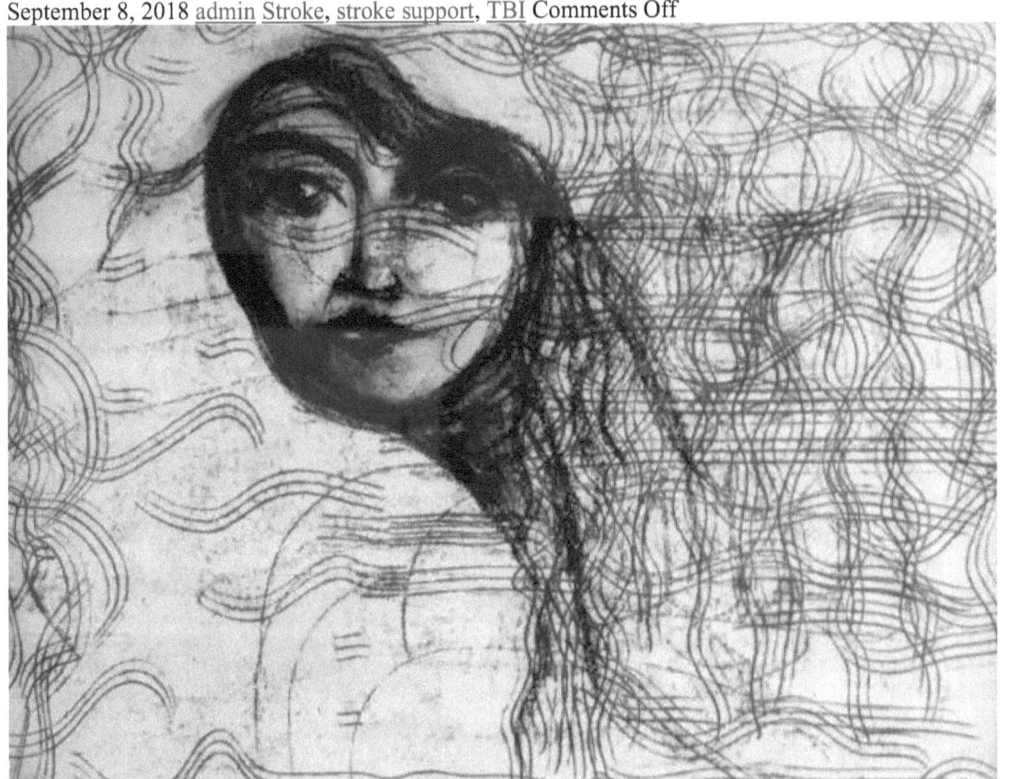

Brain Injury / Stroke and the loss of emotions. –

One of our vital brain centers that produce and regulate emotional responses is the amygdala. Precariously centered in the line of fire just above the Cerebellum, this tiny organ can be damaged irreversibly by brain injury stroke.

..

This can cause us to react with either strong out of control emotions, or with no emotions at all. Unfortunately, for too many, the effect appears to be strong emotions, such as depression, crying over any uncomfortable situation, expressions of anger or violent reactions.

..

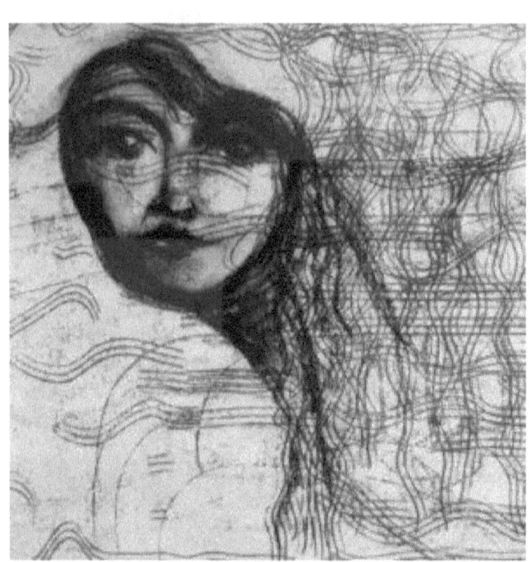

The medical solution, of course, is drug therapy to replace the actions of our amygdala to regulate the emotions. Unfortunately, these drugs cannot discriminate like our old amygdala did, and more often than not, we are turned into emotional zombies, or very close to it.

…

Talk to your Doctor! You have a right NOT to be an emotional zombie. There are many, many drugs they can select from that have varying power. Have them find the one that helps control your emotional outbursts, but does not make you a Zombie.

<u>OH HOW PAINFUL!</u>

June 10, 2018 admin Stroke, stroke support, TBI Comments Off

I cringe every time that I see canes and walkers adjusted to a height so that the victim of the adjustment (and here I will say victim), is in the obvious process of damaging themselves to the point of incurring osteoporosis. I am talking about the too short syndrome.

 OK, I am NOT a doctor, and have no medical background, but on this subject, I often wonder if medical industry has their heads in their books and are not looking at the patients.

 When your cane is too short your spine is bent to one side as you walk. Your opposite hip is thrust outward, away from the spine, and eventually tearing from the spine. Lower back pain, hip pain on the opposite hip, and sciatica pain are natural result.

 If you walk with a walker, or with two canes that are too short, and cause you to lean, you can see the obvious hunchback effect, which will result in upper back pain, middle back pain and spine pain, as well as permanently curved spine and bone spurs.

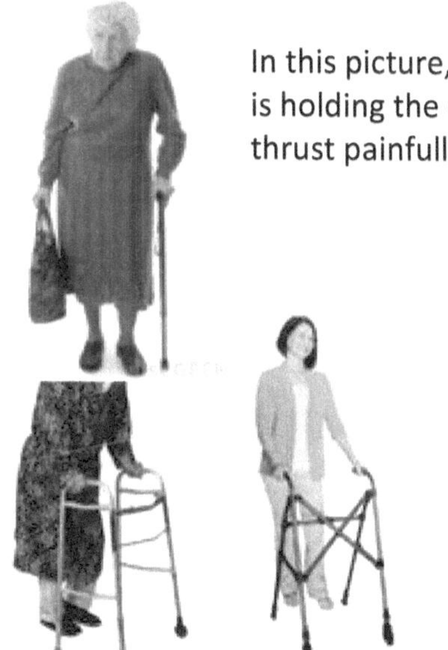

In this picture, the cane is too tall, and even though the woman is holding the cane with a bent arm, her left shoulder is still thrust painfully upward.

In these two pictures, the man has his walker adjusted too low, and is leaning forward, bending his spine, risking permanent curved spine. The lady to his right, has her walker adjusted correctly and is able to stand erect with a straight spine.

I'm not in favor on the absolute use of measurement based on hip point alone, because this does not account for the various size of a persons core (from hip to shoulder) or the length of their arms. All three of these measurements must be taken into account to properly size a mobility device.

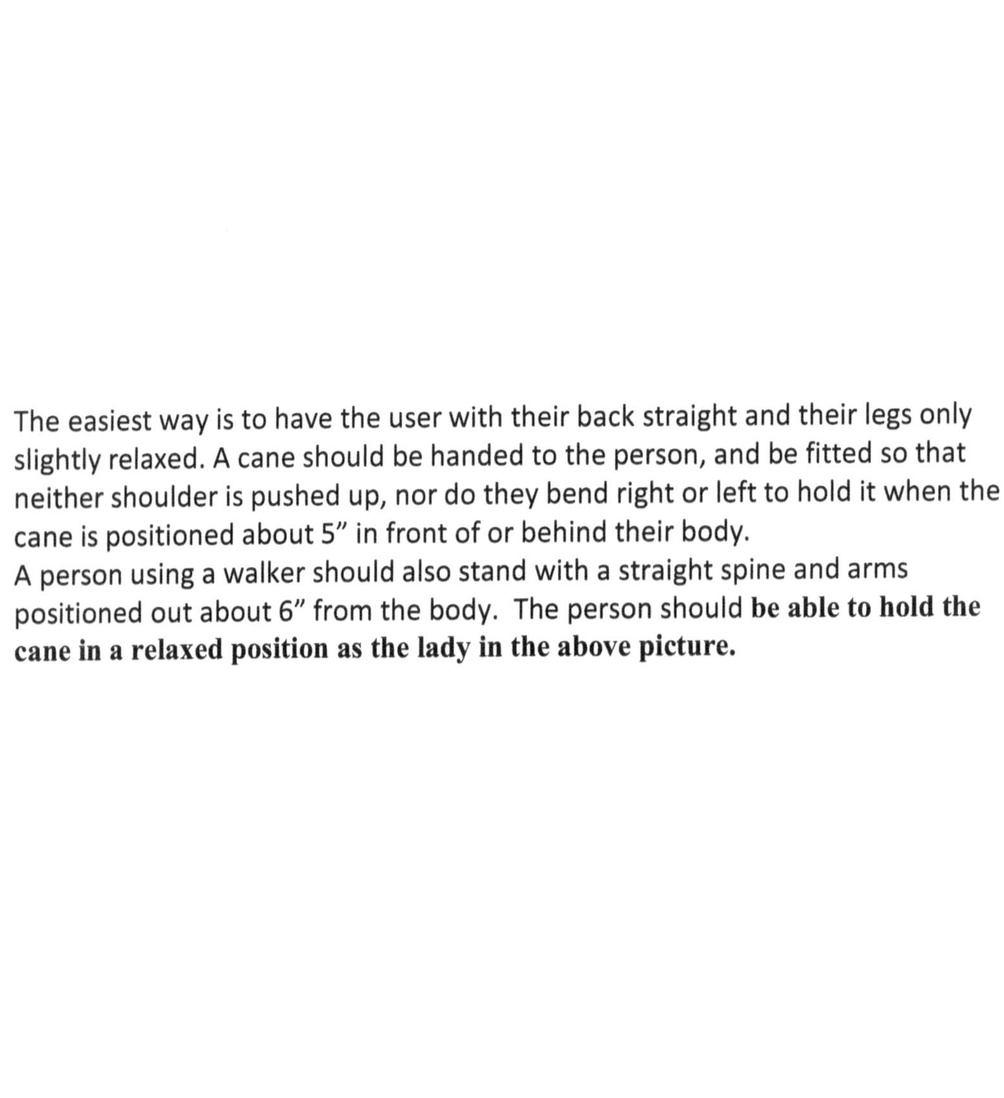

The easiest way is to have the user with their back straight and their legs only slightly relaxed. A cane should be handed to the person, and be fitted so that neither shoulder is pushed up, nor do they bend right or left to hold it when the cane is positioned about 5" in front of or behind their body.
A person using a walker should also stand with a straight spine and arms positioned out about 6" from the body. The person should **be able to hold the cane in a relaxed position as the lady in the above picture.**

Not Quite 50 First Dates...

May 15, 2018 admin Stroke, stroke support, TBI Comments Off

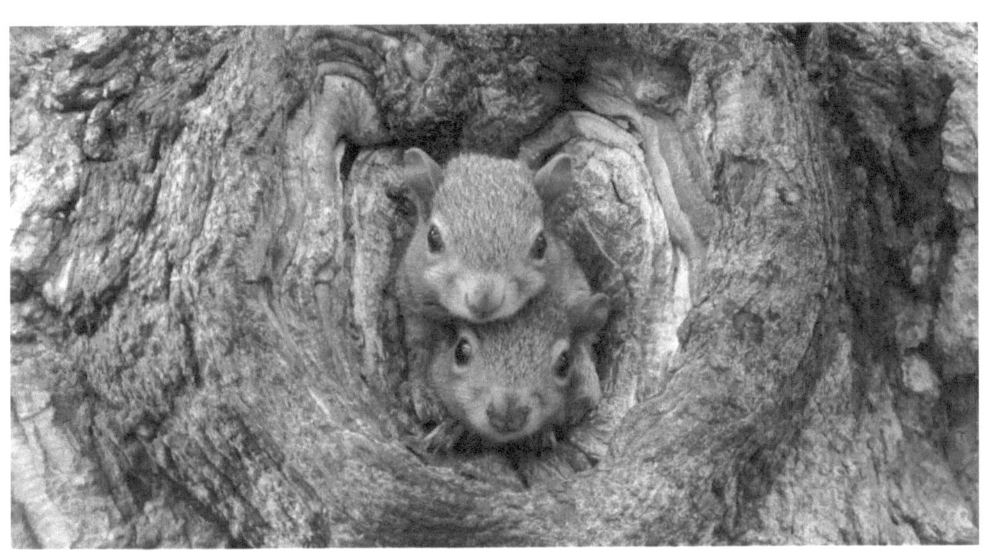

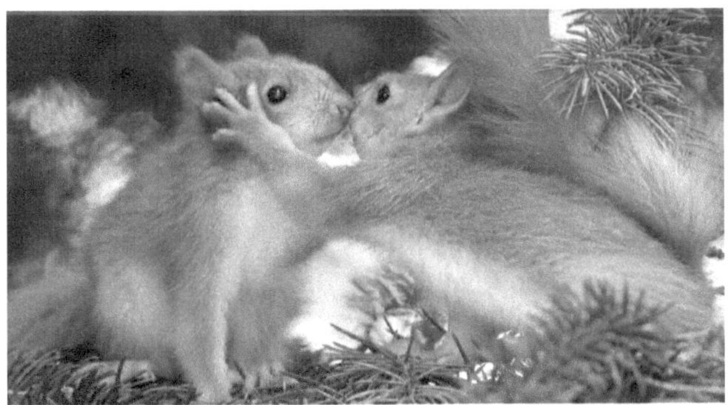

As a survivor of Brain Injury and Stroke, I know that there have been many losses to my long term memory, as well as events, feelings and people not getting posted into short term memory as they should. Normally, my days are busy enough that I don't give it a passing thought, but when I do slow down and try to reminisce about my past, I sometimes find that there is no past to reminisce about.

I don't remember my children growing up, they are now in their 30's, but what happened to their childhood, pre-teens and teen years? I look for pictures. Fortunately I was a photo hound. There are hundreds of pictures capturing wonderful moments, but how do the dots connect to each other? I finally confessed to my wife, "I love you so much, I just wish that I could remember you, I have to fall in love with you all over so many times every month, because I keep forgetting my emotional attachments.

<u>Why am I writing this?</u>

First reason, is why I write anything: to help anyone going through similar circumstances know that they are not alone, and that, even as I am experiencing this, I refuse to any answer except for "There must be more".

<u>Don't write yourself off.</u>

What *more* can you expect in the face of memory loss? One of my favorite movies before my brain injury was *50 First Dates*. A young woman with a severe brain injury has 24 hour memory that is wiped clear daily. A persistent young man refuses to give up on her and shows her increasing love each day, finally winning her as a bride. While "do-gooders" tried to not upset her and keep her safe in her memory prison, gradually her family and close friends came around to understanding that helping her grow was better than the daily trap.

I trust my support circle. They do NOT protect me by guarding my mind and memories, but encourage me to be honest, step out, ask questions, find answers, and grow. This is the MORE that we all need, people who will challenge our memories, rather than protect us in bubbles.

I hope you will find that There Is More for you too, and get the support people who will challenge your memories, and not be insulted by your Fake memories, as you try to clear everything up.

Tom Schuck

May 15, 2018 <u>admin</u> <u>Stroke</u> Comments Off

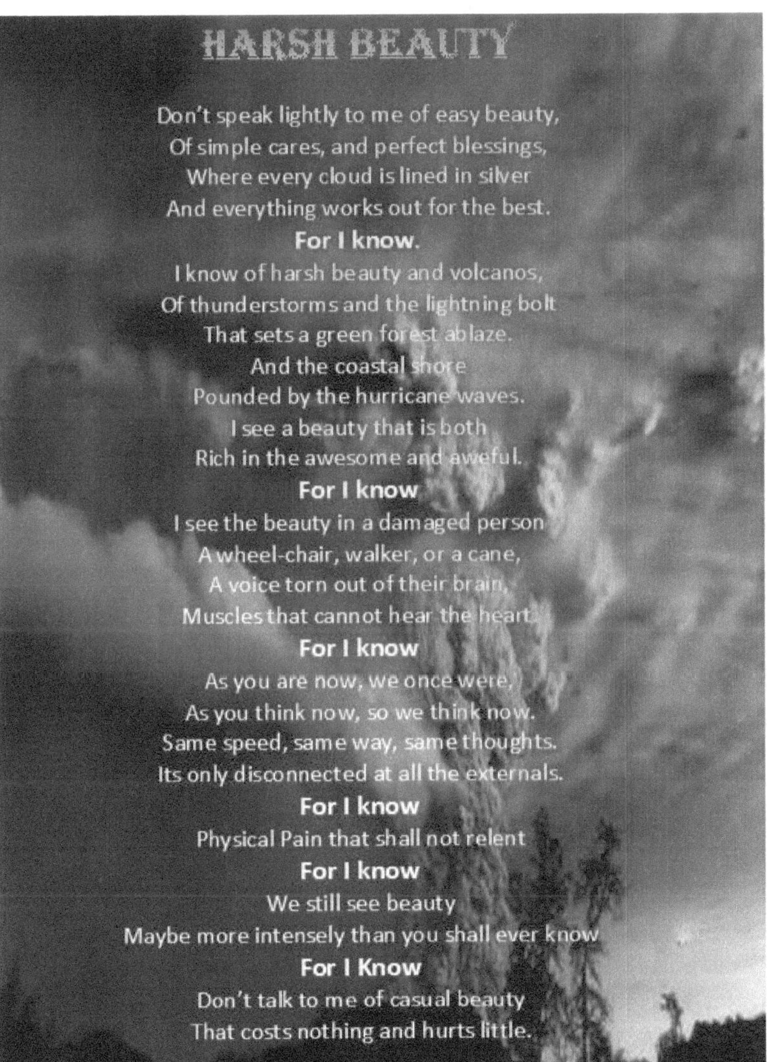

Making Money After Brain injury and Stroke

March 23, 2018 admin Stroke, stroke support, TBI Comments Off

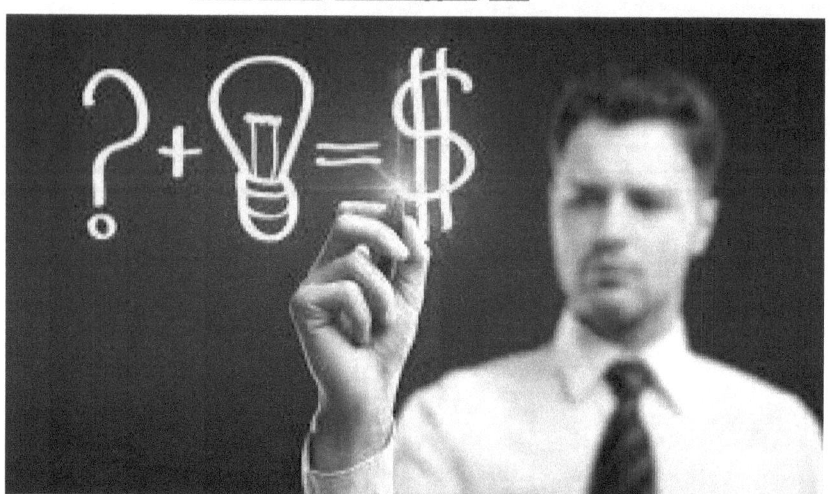

This is a popular question, so I wanted to share as much as I know about it.
The FIRST consideration is, are you on disability, and what type of
disability. Certain types of disability are filed in such a way that prevent you
"working", others that prevent you from "earning money at all", and others that
allow you to earn a very small amount of money.

CAN YOU EARN MONEY?

The problem is that since you are claiming to be "disabled", either partially or in
full, you can no longer work at the job that you used to do.

I understand that we, as survivors, have high sensitivity to crowds, noises, brightly
lit spaces, multi-tasking, and the frenetic life and work styles that we had pre-
injury and stroke. Just about every survivor that I have met, including myself,
deals with this dichotomy:

I can't do what I used to do at the pace that I used to do it.
I can do something, for much less hours per day, less days per week, yet I can do it well.
I have lost <u>some</u> of my old skills, but not all. I am still very valuable!
I also have some new skills!
Now you have to curb some of this enthusiasm with your insurance's rules and regulations. For example, I receive two types of insurance payments. SDI, which is my State Disability Payment, and will at age 65 automatically switch over to my Federal retirement benefit.
<u>MAY YOU EARN MONEY?</u>

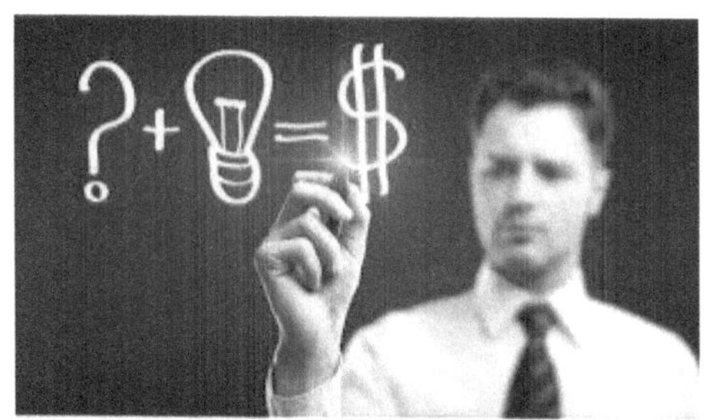

While I was working, my employer offered a private disability insurance for all employees. The employer paid a portion and I paid a portion. Though this was an optional plan, I fortunately never opted out. This supplemental insurance has very tight restrictions. It is in force to age 65, and pays 65% of pre-disability income. The two major restrictions are, I am not allowed to even earn one cent as long as I am collecting this insurance, and second, I must be willing to take medical exams as proof of my continued disability.
With State SDI and even retirement the rules vary, from zero-no-tolerance, to just allowing you to earn just over 1,000 per month. If you earn more than the rules allow, you will penalized by deductions in your insurance or retirement coverage.
What about earning money "under the table"?
Don't do this. You can possibly claim ignorance or an accounting error for incorrectly reported expenses, but the IRS is UNFORGIVING for unreported income. There is so much risk in doing this. Just watch TV.
Ok, so you've done your homework, and you want to work, now what.
<u>HOW TO EARN MONEY?</u>
The key to the American economy has always been:
Find a need. Is there something that people hate doing, or put off doing forever.
Create a need. Convince people that they are doing something the hard way
Fill the need. Be the person or company to solve the need that people have.

I can tell you that there is an endless list of things that people and companies do that they really don't want to do or hire a full time person for.

But then you want to think about, what are my skills? What are the things that I can really do?

- ➢ Document processor
    - o "send me your documents, I will scan at only $xx.xx per page and return your documents and all documents on PDF
    - o Possible Clients
        - ▪ Individuals
        - ▪ Small offices – doctors
        - ▪ Medium offices
    - o "send me your photographs, I will scan all at high resolution
    - o Possible clients
        - ▪ Individuals
        - ▪ Small offices
    - o Database processor
    - o Send me your paper documents
        - ▪ I will create a searchable excel sheet with mail merge
        - ▪ I will enter everything into a database
- ➢ I will come into office for 2 weeks, 2 hours per day
    - o I will type all your paper into you're a database
    - o I will type all your data into excel
- ➢ Petsitter
    - o You must get license for this
- ➢ Assembler
    - o I can assemble any small items that you need
- ➢ Work at a Charitable organization
    - o Most charitable organizations recognize your limitations
- ➢ Willing to work-share
- ➢ Use your existing skills

How Long until I am well?

Your brain continues making fine tuning correction and re-pathing around damaged areas to enable as many lost abilities to be returned to you.
It is impossible for the first 3 to 5 years to make any conclusions about your final state of healing. It is also critical during these years to utilize as much Physical Therapy, Vision Therapy, Speech Therapy, etc., as you possibly need.

This section is for those who are entering the extended stage after 3-5 years of treatment, when it appears that a group of deficits from the original brain injury or stroke have settled into a pattern of permanence.

Before I continue, I will give some generalized and unsupportable statistics. Nevertheless, anecdotally, they are the best statistics that I have read or heard from various resources:
Note: These apply to individuals below the age of 80 who have had a first time brain injury or stroke.

- About 60% of all individuals will survive with zero to little noticeable deficits, that do not impede quality of life or quantity of activity.
- About 38% of all individuals will survive will have some degree of deficits that do impede there quality of life and quantity of activity.
  - Of that 38% group:
    - About 50% will return to some kind of limited work
    - About 60% will be able to drive, but probably will self-limit to daylight hours
    - About 33% will experience symptoms or deficits that often interrupt or cancel plans or events.

<u>Putting *OLD ME* skills into *NEW ME* ABILITIES</u>

Most caregivers and support programs focus around creating all-new programs that completely ignore the history and background to the individual. Not only is this damaging to the individual's self-worth, but it devalues their entire past.

In addition to focusing on long term goals that benefit and strengthen the "new me", shift some of the focus to finding opportunities where the "old me" can be expressed through fun activities for a short period of time. As long as the deficits (pain, vertigo, speech problems, confusion, ambulatory devices, etc.) will allow, creatively discover anything that can be done to provide the survivor with experiences similar to what they enjoyed in their "old me" life.

These experiences, or what I called "visits" to what they used to be or used to do, or events they used to enjoy, are designed to allow the "old normal" to happily resurface for a brief time.   They may provide the survivor a sense of joy and accomplishment.

Family members and counselors could encourage the survivor to remember what some of these were, so that together they can craft the opportunities to let it happen. The survivor may need to be reminded that since these are only visits with the "old me", and not healings, that there will always be an end to each experience or "visit".

Here are some ideas from my personal experiences of "old normal" activities and emotions that can lead to these momentary successes:

<u>**Fluid Motion.**</u>
There's a normal excitement on the part of caregivers to think of the great many
wonderful "new normal" opportunities: therapy pools, walking, yoga, etc. But
what I am suggesting is discovering meaningful activities of fluid motion from
their "old me" and then crafting ways for how they might be reproduced or
mimicked for short periods of time. This can become more challenging and more
rewarding for those whose existing motion is now limited by the need for
ambulatory devices.

Personal Examples:
1. Before my injury, my wife and I loved to ballroom dance. We were pretty
   good as a couple. My wife still takes me ballroom dancing, I cannot balance
   without her supporting me, therefore I cannot dance with others, but
   dancing together has been something that we have enjoyed for years.
   Now, she has to support my balance, and be an encouragement as I try to
   do my best
2. I love water sports. Initially, I refused to sell my kayak for 3 years following
   my initial brain injury, but finally realizing that my balance made it
   dangerous for me to contInue, I ended up selling it and all the gear. But
   very shortly afterwards, I found an organization in my state (CT) that
   provides sailing experiences and education to persons with brain injuries in
   Long Island Sound.

For others, it may be golf, or some other sports that can be replicated or
mimicked if at all possible, for whatever brief period of time. A survivor can play
many games from a wheel chair, you can even choreograph baseball or football
where all the players may only walk.

<u>**Forgetting pain.**</u>

Forgetting pain does not replace the therapy of reducing pain through medications and other means, rather it is filling the senses with delightful stimulation that allows the survivor to forget their pain, even for brief moments.

- Laughter: For some, forgetting pain may be as easy as remembering what used to cause joy, laughter, silliness, delight. Work with the survivor to remember and explore those activities that delighted or consumed them. Then develop environments to help them have periods of time like that again.

- Physical Touch. Perhaps the most significant way to forget pain for a moment is through human touch. When a survivor is especially needy, or unable to control their bodily functions, friends and family members may discover that they are treating their loved one with a patient/caregiver mentality. Over time, the person providing care can be overcome with routine chores, and become too exhausted to take time to love. The survivor, meanwhile, wishes for and needs, the loving touch and friend so much more that they do the physical care that they receive. There are several support groups for caregivers, physical and on-line, if you find yourself in this situation.

- Shouldn't Have to Ask. Spouses and family members often have little insight into the severe emotional unbalance caused by TBI and similar neurological diseases. The often excessive displays of need for affection that is produced by damage to the brain is no more controllable, nor the fault of the survivor than was the injury or disease. It is unreasonable to expect that a survivor reacts with all the normal social conventions, especially when they are in pain, dizziness, or brain confusion. If a caregiver sees a survivor motioning a need or desire for affection or care, and does not respond ONLY because the caregiver is demanding that the survivor asks in a normal manner, I suggest that is an uncharitable nature, bordering on abuse.

Challenging the brain.

There are many excellent new normal brain challenging activities for the survivor, software programs, apps, adult coloring books and other activities, but again, I am looking backward, what brain-challenges did the survivor enjoy before their incident? Crosswords? Puzzles? Soduko?

For me, what used to challenge my brain was writing software programs and mathematical algorithms. Also, I loved creative writing, such as this little book, but did not get much time to do any. Now, I find concentrating on software algorithms impossible and doing simple math such as calculating the tip on a restaurant bill nearly impossible. But, with the help of Dragon Speech and other great software tools, I get a great deal of satisfaction writing even though my eyes and fingers are still uncooperative.

Challenging the brain can take on many other forms depending on what the "old me" experiences were for each individual. There are many "new normal" activities to challenge the brain that have been devised by the medical community and caregivers over the years, and these are excellent and appreciated therapies. However, again, I am suggesting discovering with us what we felt challenged our brain, and then helping us to repeat or mimic some of those activities.

<u>**Feeling valued and needed.**</u>
Pain, confusion, or being confined to ambulatory devices or other medical devices are inhibitors to the survivor's feeling needed and valued. A survivor with a brain injury is not, and never will be the same as, a person who has been living with lifetime mental health symptoms.

In almost every case, a survivor's psyche is fully functional, just as was it was the moment before their accident or disease set in. A caregiver's frustration at the inability of their loved one to get their thoughts out quickly or clearly, is nothing compared to the survivor's frustration of trying to vocalize thought.

The "old normal" included many ways that every survivor in healthy relationships were able to feel value and needed. They could do good deeds for others, or perform special tasks at work that would gain respect and admiration. However, within the context of their "new normal", admiration may only come for their ability to put up with pain and circumstances.

<u>**Family examples:**</u>
1. Husbands may experience crushing memories of their "old me" roles around the house, especially if his identity was wrapped up in 'typical western society male roles'. In life after brain injury or stroke, the husband may be unable to perform or accomplish many of these roles. The wife or children may not only take charge, but prevent him from trying. The wife may offer all sorts of "new me" experiences for her husband without realizing that she is offering pony rides to a war horse. The war horse will do the pony rides, but the couple should look for ways to help recreate old normal experiences for the husband to enjoy.

2. Wives will have memories of their "old me" roles also. All of the things that she used to do that she valued as part of her identity such as making the house a home for her and her husband, having a valuable career, home business, or community advocate. Now, feeling set aside and useless, she watches as her husband does all these things instead. The couple should look for ways to enjoy "old normal" experiences.

Medicines and Weight Gain

There are too many medications that treat the aftermath of stroke and brain injury that include that side affect "may cause weight gain". Most of the preferred neurological pain medications are infamous for this side effect. I recommend working with your neurologist early on to try different medications for neurological pain.

One of the top rated, most commonly prescribed is "Lyrica (generic: pregabalin)". It is a very good medication at treating neuralgia (nerve pain), but has an extremely high (anecdotal) rate of rapid weight gain in many patients.

Another commonly used, well tolerated alternative is "Neurontin (generic: gabapentin) ". Also good at treating neuralgia (nerve pain), but also has a high (anecdotal) rate of weight gain in many patients.

If you experience any unsatisfactory side effects, don't hesitate to discuss these with your neurologist and find out what other recommendations they may make.

Finding "New Me" Hobbies

Rule #1. Don't be afraid to experiment.

In the theme song for Zootopia "Try Everything", the repeating phrase "I keep on making those new mistakes" is good advice for rebuilding your life.

In my old life, I was a well-paid and well-esteemed project manager and IT executive, situated handsomely on the corporate ladder, until…..

After my brain injury, I did go back to work, for about 18 months, struggling to prove to myself and others that I was unaffected. Then, after about 18 months, I incurred a second stroke directly related to the brain injury. I continued to try to drive, to try to work, but it was obvious that my processing skills and mental stamina were very poor. To the relief of everyone, my neurologist determined that I should be put on permanent disability.

Now I had the struggle of who was I? I was no longer a project manager or IT executive, and I could not even write a single line of software code, something that I had been doing for over 30 years.

I tried puzzles, origami, oil painting. Nothing worked.

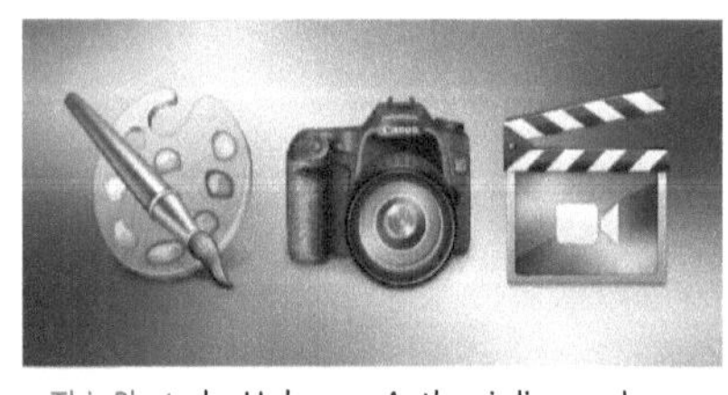

I purchased expensive camera equipment to photograph birds. Birds are annoying, they won't stand still. I started photographing nature, then honed in on squirrels. Meanwhile, I started writing. I also purchased a 3D printer and started designing small and useful items. I finally felt busy again.

But all of this required many set-backs, frustrations and buying equipment that ended up in the junk pile, because I thought it would be suitable for me. I kept making new mistakes.

I now have a well-defined "New Me" that looks nothing like the "old me", but is as fun and enjoyable and even more so, than the old me ever was.

Avoiding Stimulating Situations

In the Chapter "Why didn't they tell me this", I covered several of the common major stimulating situations, but I want to explore them a little more in depth here.

1. Bright Lights, Florescent Lights.
    a. There are several temperatures of light that are measured in "Kelvins".
        i. At the lowest end, is the Yellow light below 5000k. This Dim light is often used at night to mimic the color of moon light, and ranges from bright yellow to dingy brown. Low kelvin light is easy to move around in, or watch TV in, but is inappropriate for reading or detailed eye-work. Unfortunately, many banks of florescent lights often emit in this low color range. Rather than replacing low kelvin bulbs with white bulbs, many buildings just increase the number of yellow bulbs. This leads to (anecdotally) to sleepiness, and poor concentration.
        ii. In the middle is White light, about 6-7500 kelvins, which is similar to daytime sun. Good for indoor lighting, but can be too intense at the higher end of the scale for office work.
        iii. At the top of the scale is blue light, kelvins (10,000-11,000k). This is NOT blue colored light, bluish white. Because of its brilliance its intensity can be lowered dramatically, and it will still be effective. Anecdotally, I find this color, tuned to lower intensity, to be the best tolerated by survivors as a background light in reading, and working on the computer.

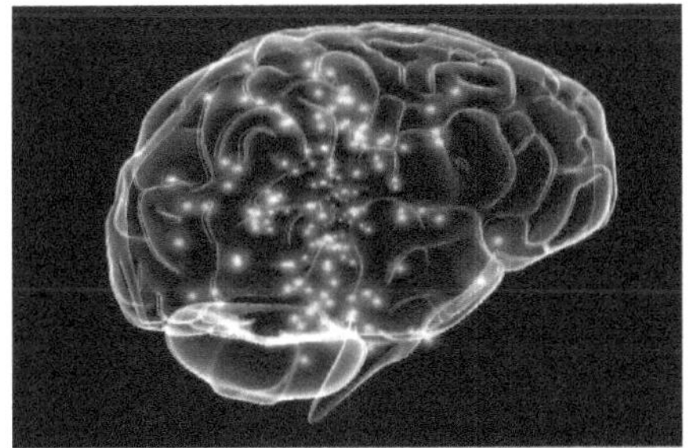

a. There are also several delivery methods of lighting
    i. Halogen and other industrial – Brilliant, usually Yellow
    ii. Incandescent. The standard household bulb of the 50s – now, this inexpensive toss away bulb mixes economics with good light delivery. Can be found in Yellow or White.
    iii. Fluorescent. A Standard in many offices and garages and annoying at end of cycle due to its pulsing effect. This light works through a constant pulsing effect, which is normally unnoticeable, but for some reason, individuals with brain injury, stroke, concussion, etc., appear to have a greater sensitivity. Fluorescent bulbs are not a good choice around individuals who have experienced these situations.
    iv. LED. This new light delivery, has a standard bright color of bluish white, and it can be easily controlled by power delivery for intensity. It can be colored at the manufacturer with many artificial colors. Bundled together, LED lights are now used in headlights on cars, office lighting, house lightbulbs and more. Their excellent color and tone and resistance to visible pulsing makes them a great choice.
b. Instead of annoying office or artificial lighting try filtered sun-light through a window with blinds or drapes
c. Wear sunglasses indoors and out. Don't worry about looking too cool.
d. Reduce the brightness of your computer, laptop or tablet screen.

2. Interior Sunglasses
    a. Try driver's sunglasses (the yellow lens) to remove inside glare and reduce light.
    b. If that does not work, then try darker brown glasses or glasses to your style

3. Remove yourself from noisy conversations. If you find that being in the presence of hearing multiple conversations taking place at one time in near proximity overtaxes your brain:
    e. Always bring along ear plugs
    f. If needed, bring along noise cancelling ear buds to plug into your cell phone.
4. Offer alternatives to overcrowded venues: If you find that being in large crowded situations overtaxes your brain.
    g. When plans are being made to go somewhere, offer your suggestion to go somewhere less crowded

Personal Countermeasures

This may sound odd, but I found that my wife and my friends enjoy the extra time that they get to spend at events or outings without the interruption of my need to break it off.

By this time, my wife and friends have understood and somewhat emphasize that there is no selfishness in my statement, "I am done, I need to leave". It is simply a statement of unresolvable fact. But I have found a countermeasure that allows me to satisfactorily "implode" and escape the stimulating environments without leaving.

After observing how often many pre-teens and teens can tune-out by reading or playing a video game, I discovered that I, with my brain injury, could also bring along a book, audio book, video game, etc. and completely tune-out everything around me.

My wife and friends do not comment when I pull out my iPad to listen to or read my book or play my game. They understand that I am giving everyone else more time together, but separating myself for the moment. If works great once it has been explained.

<u>Role changes</u>

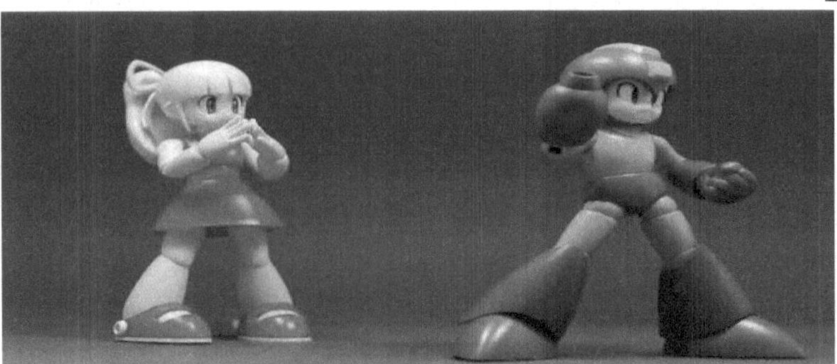

Once again, this covers a broad range of survivors' experiences, your personal experience may be far less complicated.

Generally, this hits home in the home, especially where the family was structured around perceived "roles" for the husband, wife, older and younger children of each gender.

- Those that prided themselves on being in the workforce, bringing home the lion's share of the paycheck, and sustaining the family, feel helpless and often worthless as their spouses and other family members have to take on extra burden of jobs and extra work just to pay family bills.
- Those that prided themselves on maintaining and managing the chaos of a successful home schedule, mixing domestic responsibilities with some outside work, will feel the pain of usefulness taken away as others cook for them, clean for them, possibly feed, and chauffer them all around.

Other than the stroke or brain injury survivor, the family members are often unaware of how this dynamic affects the heart of the survivors.

Mostly what IS needed is NOT just verbal reassurances, but giving tasks that the survivor can successfully accomplish. This will provide the survivor a sense of fulfillment and participation in the family dynamic.

Provide specific tasks that the survivor can do, or can lead, based on their current abilities. At first, make sure that you set them up for success, then make the tasks a little more challenging where failure is possible unless they ask for help.

<u>There Is More</u>

I really hope that within this book you picked up the information that you need for your journey.

Please check my other books on brain injury only on Amazon, Paperback and Kindle.

A View From the Inside: A Survivors Perspective of Brain Injury and Stroke

https://www.amazon.com/dp/1508881456/

Search for Spiritual Meaning After Brain Injury/Stroke: Building a new me

https://www.amazon.com/ dp/B00U0SD4Z0/

Please check out our website at

www.thereismoremeeting.com

If you are visiting the Hartford, CT area and would like to check out our meetings on the 2nd and 4th Fridays, please e-mail first wincss@yahoo.com for current locations and direction.